About the Author

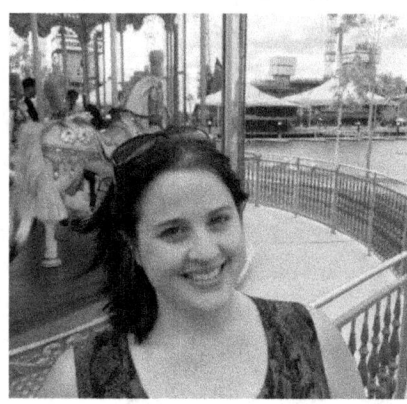

Thanks so much for purchasing "Healing with Astaxanthin". My name is Jennifer Matthews and I am also known as Naturopath Jen. I am a qualified Naturopath, Law of Attraction Practitioner, Spiritual Life Coach and Self-Empowerment Educator. I have spent the last decade researching and spending thousands of dollars on my own personal development, as well as previously hosting multiple podcasts and blogs in the areas of health, wellness, mindset and spirituality.

I am now the founder and developer of the "Superconscious Success" Platform and the "Ask Naturopath Jen" Brand.

To learn more about myself and my journey (as it is quite an extensive read), please visit my personal site: http://www.spiritualcoachjenmatthews.com, where I delve into my purpose for writing these books and creating these brands and all the products/services (both free and paid) that can help you.

PREFACE

Are you a fitness fanatic that is not recovering from your workouts? Are you dealing with inflammatory conditions that leave you in constant pain and discomfort? If so, then Astaxanthin may be just what you are looking for.

Astaxanthin is a potently powerful nutrient commonly found in seafood and algae but is also able to be found in supplement form if you know exactly what to look for.

ABOUT THE BOOK

Healing with Astaxanthin is the fourth book in the ANJ Series because it is a nutrient that I am absolutely fascinated with and I take myself every day. With so many people suffering from painful inflammatory conditions like arthritis and autoimmune irregularity, I thought it was not only an important book to write, but also one that I find quite interesting.

OTHER BOOKS IN THIS SERIES

(All Available in Amazon under Naturopath Jen)

MSM Uncovered

Magnificent Magnesium

The Acne Solution

DISCLAIMER

Please note that the information given in this book is for informational purposes only and is not intended to replace the advice of your health practitioner. If you experience symptoms that you are concerned with please refer to your practitioner for further information...

****

SECTION 1 – INTRO TO ASTAXANTHIN

****

Chapter #1 - Astaxanthin Basics

****

What is Astaxanthin?

It is likely that you have heard about the antioxidants beta-carotene (found in orange fruits and vegetables) and lutein (found in leafy green vegetables). But you may not have heard about the most powerful antioxidant of them all - Astaxanthin...

Astaxanthin differs from many of the other antioxidants because:

- It is much more powerful - Astaxanthin is over 6000 times stronger than Vitamin C, 550 times stronger than Vitamin E and 2000 times stronger than resveratrol and quercetin. To learn more about this, please check out Chapter #2.
- It remains active for a longer period of time - Due to the fact that astaxanthin has a massive surplus of free electrons, its antioxidant capacity will last a lot longer. Once it has donated the electrons to neutralize the free radicals, it will eliminate the excess energy as heat.
- It can handle multiple free radicals at any given time - Most antioxidants can only handle one free radical at a time, but astaxanthin can handle up to 19 free radicals at once.
- It positions itself across the entire cell membrane, which is unlike any other carotenoid:
- A portion will attach to the exterior of the cell (offers protection from free radicals outside of the cell);
- A portion will attach to the interior (offers protection inside where there are free radicals being generated); and
- A portion across the entire lipid layer (to protect against lipid peroxidation).
- It is able to cross the blood-brain barrier and blood-retinal barrier, therefore creating anti-inflammatory protection to the brain and the eyes. Most antioxidants are unable to do this (apart from resveratrol).

Why is Astaxanthin so good for you?

Astaxanthin is a powerful antioxidant and anti-inflammatory, which is particularly known for its benefits with skin health and eye health. As most conditions are caused from inflammation, Astaxanthin is very effective at helping to treat inflammatory conditions.

To learn more about Antioxidants and Inflammation, please see Chapter #2 on "Primary Functions of Astaxanthin".

Signs of Antioxidant Deficiency

When your body doesn't have enough antioxidants, the deficiency can cause free radicals to roam within the cells leading to cell damage. This cell damage leads to changes in the DNA, which can contribute to a whole host of conditions such as:

1. Alzheimers Disease;
2. Cancer;
3. Eye Disease;
4. Heart Disease;
5. Parkinson's Disease; and
6. Rheumatoid Arthritis.

Nutritional Sources of Astaxanthin...

When talking about most nutrients, I will always say that I prefer you to obtain that nutrient from food first, and then take supplements when required.

However, in the case of Astaxanthin, I will say that supplements are actually much more powerful than nutrition alone.

That is not to say, however that you shouldn't try to obtain as much as you can from food, but if you are really wanting to get the effects of this amazing antioxidant, then consider supplementation.

For instance, you would need to consume over a pound of salmon every day just to get 4mg of Astaxanthin. Far more than most can tolerate.

However, I will first go into the food sources of Astaxanthin:

Astaxanthin is the deep red, fat soluble pigment which is found in many different sources throughout nature.

If you are wanting to include more astaxanthin rich foods in your diets, then try to incorporate more of the following:

Fish/Seafood
1. Wild Pacific Sockeye Salmon (highest concentration);
2. Krill;
3. Red Trout;
4. Shrimp;
5. Crab;
6. Lobster.

Although all salmon contains some Astaxanthin, it is important to remember that wild caught salmon is 400 times richer in this antioxidant than the farm caught variety.

When deciding what food to eat, the quality of the food is very important. Wild caught fish ingest microalgae from the sea, but farm raised fish consume synthetic astaxanthin from petrochemicals. Synthetic astaxanthin is 20-50 times weaker in antioxidants than the natural sources.

Algae

Astaxanthin is created by a micro-algae called Haematococcus Pluvialis. The Astaxanthin within this algae acts as a force field around it during times of stress, allowing it to live for 40+ years without food or water.

Yeast

On top of these sources, there is a form of yeast, known as Xanthophyllomyces dendrorhous (Phaffia) which is rich in astaxanthin. However, this is generally not used for human consumption.

Why Don't We Get Enough Antioxidants In Our Diet?

There are many reasons why you may not have enough supply of antioxidants and why astaxanthin may be useful for you...

1. **Ageing** - As you get older, your body makes less of your naturally produced antioxidants (i.e. Glutathione) and therefore an external supply may be warranted.
2. **Smoking** - People regularly exposed to cigarette smoke will experience greater free radical production, therefore requiring more antioxidants.
3. **Alcohol** - Studies (48) have shown that alcohol consumption can decrease a multitude of antioxidants, such as alpha tocopherol, ascorbic acid and selenium.
4. **Digestive Issues** - If you are not digesting food properly then you will also not be absorbing the nutrients you require, including the important antioxidant zinc.
5. **Vegetarians/Vegans** - As vegetables are not a great source of zinc, vegetarians and vegans will often be low in antioxidants.

Supplemental Forms of Astaxanthin

Astaxanthin is one nutrient that I suggest you get from supplementation as well as nutrition. Although you can find it in fish, you would need to eat a lot of it to get enough of the benefits.

Ensure that when you are searching for the perfect Astaxanthin supplement, you make sure it comes from Marine Microalgae (H Pluvialis) and not cheap sources made from various synthetic petrochemicals.

Astaxanthin from microalgae contains 40,000 parts per million, as opposed to 40 ppm in Salmon, 120 ppm in Krill and 1200 ppm in Shrimp.

My recommended source of astaxanthin can be found at http://www.asknaturopathjen.com/store

Storage of Astaxanthin...

There are a number of factors that can affect the quality and level of astaxanthin:

4. Long term exposure to air;
5. Long term exposure to light;
6. Contact with heat.

Storing your food in airtight containers in dark places and minimizing the time you cook, may help reduce astaxanthin degradation. This is why it is important to not overcook your fish/seafood and why sashimi can be so good for you (as long as it is from a safe source).

Best Time to Take Astaxanthin...

There is no specific time when it is best to take Astaxanthin. But, as Astaxanthin is fat soluble, you must ensure you take it with fat.

Dosage and Toxicity of Astaxanthin...

Thankfully, Astaxanthin is one of the least toxic nutrients you can take. It is able to be taken safely with most medications and has absolutely no known record of toxicity. However, because of its effectiveness, it may require you reducing your other medications. Please see the section on contraindications to figure out if this applies to you.

If you take high doses of up to 50mg per day you might get a slight orange tinge due to the nutrient becoming stored in your fat tissues. However, this is no cause for alarm and all you need to do is go off it for a few days to a week and then start again at a lower dose.

The recommended dosage is between 12 and 16mg per day, PLUS any food sources you would like to consume.

Supplements to take with Astaxanthin

Because astaxanthin is a fat-soluble antioxidant, it is a great idea to take it with some form of fat. You can either take it with a high fat meal, or use the following supplements:

1. Fish Oil;

2. Vitamin C;

3. Ginkgo Biloba;

4. MCT Oil;

5. Coconut Oil;

6. Flax Oil.

Cautions/Contraindications/Medicine Interactions

1.   Although astaxanthin is an incredibly safe supplement to take, there are a few things to keep in mind:

2.   If you have diabetes or hypo-glycemia and you are using astaxanthin just remember that you may need to adjust your medications. Astaxanthin is very effective at lowering blood glucose levels and improving insulin sensitivity.

3.   If you have hypertension and you are taking drugs or supplements to lower it, be cautious as you may need to lower your dosage. Astaxanthin is very effective at lowering blood pressure.

4.   Be careful if you are on any 5 alpha reductase inhibitors, calcium salts, drugs that affect bleeding heart medications, hormonal agents, immunosuppressants and rofecoxib as astaxanthin may interact with it.

5.   If you are on any medications, check with your pharmacy or medical practitioner to see if they use the cytochrome P450 enzyme system, as astaxanthin may interfere with the way the body processes the drugs.

Chapter #2 - Primary Functions of Astaxanthin

****

There are 2 main functions that Astaxanthin plays within the body, which explains it's amazing benefits:

1.   Potent Antioxidant
2.   Potent Anti-Inflammatory

Potent Antioxidant

What Are Antioxidants?

Antioxidants are molecules within your body that are used to inhibit oxidation of another molecule. One theory is that how many antioxidants you have available will determine how quickly you age.

Free Radicals are highly reactive metabolites that are naturally produced by your body in response to metabolism, exercise, energy production, inflammation and even exposure to a variety of environmental toxins (i.e. Cigarettes, Sunlight and Chemicals).

These free radicals can damage your DNA and cell structure by stealing electrons from the proteins within your body and as these molecules steal from one another they then become a new free radical and cause even more damage within your body.

Antioxidants are there to give up their own electrons to feed the free radicals so that this oxidative damage does not occur, without becoming a free radical itself.

Why is Astaxanthin called "The Super Antioxidant"?

Astaxanthin is truly a super antioxidant. If you were to look at the ORAC (Oxygen Radical Absorbance Capacity) Score, you would see that it is in fact higher than so many other super foods. The higher the ORAC score, the higher the antioxidant capacity.

Astaxanthin	28,222
Ginger	14,840
Pomegranate	10,500
Black Beans	8,040
Garlic	5,346
Broccoli	2,809
Spinach	1,515
Olive Oil	1,150
Banana	879
Tomato	700

Plus, in terms of other supplements, you will notice that it also outranks them...

1. 65 times more powerful than Vitamin C as a free radical scavenger and 6000 times stronger than Vitamin C as a singlet oxygen quencher;
2. 54 times more powerful than Beta Carotene as a free radical scavenger;
3. 14 times more powerful than Vitamin E as a free radical scavenger and 550 times more powerful than Vitamin E as a singlet oxygen quencher;
4. 800 times stronger than Co Q10 as a singlet oxygen quencher.

Please Note:
Singlet Oxygen is the most reactive of the two forms of free radicals. A Singlet Oxygen Quencher is one which is powerful at eliminating these species...

Potent Anti-Inflammatory

What is Inflammation?

Inflammation is a protective response by the body when there is any sort of trauma, bacteria, viruses or other physiological changes that are not beneficial to the organism.

Inflammation is a natural process that occurs so as to trigger the immune system to heal the injury. The process of inflammation is quite interesting:

1. The arterioles will dilate and new capillaries and venular beds will open up in that area. This causes an accelerated flow of blood, which leads to the common inflammatory symptoms of heat and redness.
2. Next is when there is increased permeability in the circulation, causing fluid to leak out into the extravascular fluid compartment. This leads to inflammatory edema (swelling).
3. Then the immune system takes charge. Leukocytes, Neutrophils and Macrophages all play a part to neutralize the foreign particles by a process known as phagocytosis.

Inflammation is not bad in itself. It is when you are chronically inflamed that your endocrine system starts to go into overdrive, as does your immune system.

Main Types of Inflammation

1. Acute Inflammation - Sudden Onset causing heat, redness, swelling, pain and loss of function.
2. Sub-acute Inflammation - Condition in-between acute and chronic inflammation.
3. Chronic Inflammation - Prolonged and persistent inflammation marked by new connective tissue formation.

Why Is Astaxanthin such a great Anti-Inflammatory?

When your body is chronically inflamed, your immune system will go into overdrive. After an injury or attack, as is the case with inflammation, a number of mediators (such as prostaglandins, TNF, interleukins and nitric oxide) are released.

Anti-Inflammatory drugs work by limiting the production of these prostaglandins and therefore they ease swelling and pain. Unfortunately, anti-inflammatory drugs have side effects that can be unpleasant and unnatural for the body.

Thankfully, there are anti-inflammatory foods that can ease inflammation by gently inhibiting these mediators, so as to gradually calm the system. There are also anti-inflammatory supplements which can be of great benefit. Astaxanthin is one of these.

Astaxanthin suppresses anti-inflammatory mediators such as tumour necrosis factor alpha, nitric oxide, COX-1 enzyme and COX-2 enzyme.

Although Astaxanthin is not quite as effective as many of the most powerful pharmaceutical anti-inflammatories and it takes a little longer to take effect it can still be a better option as it does not come with all the negative side effects of common pharmaceuticals. Astaxanthin is found to be one of the most powerful natural anti-inflammatories in nature.

Because of its anti-inflammatory properties, you may find it helpful in treating inflammatory conditions such as:

1. Tennis Elbow;
2. Carpal Tunnel Syndrome;
3. Rheumatoid Arthritis; and
4. Post Exercise Soreness.

What are other great Anti-Inflammatories?

Supplements

1.MSM;
2.Fish Oil;
3.Quercetin;
4.Curcumin;
5.Resveratrol;
6.Ginger;
7.Alpha Lipoic Acid;
8.Zinc.

Foods

Leafy Vegetables - 1 cup includes these anti-inflammatories:

639% Daily Value of Vitamin K;
60% Daily Value of Vitamin A;
42% Daily Value of Vitamin C.

Bok Choy - 1 cup includes these anti-inflammatories:

64% Daily Value of Vitamin K;
59% Daily Value of Vitamin A;
40% Daily Value of Vitamin C.

Celery - 1 cup includes these anti-inflammatories:

37% Daily Value of Vitamin K;
9% Daily Value of Vitamin A;
8% Daily Value of Potassium;
5% Daily Value of Vitamin C.

Beets - 1 cup includes these anti-inflammatories:

34% Daily Value of Folate;
28% Daily Value of Manganese;
15% Daily Value of Potassium;
10% Daily Value of Magnesium.

Blueberries - 1 cup includes these anti-inflammatories:

36% Daily Value of Vitamin K;
25% Daily Value of Vitamin C;
25% Daily Value of Manganese.

Broccoli - 1 cup includes these anti-inflammatories:

254% Daily Value of Vitamin K;
135% Daily Value of Vitamin C;
53% Daily Value of Chromium;
42% Daily Value of Folate;
18% Daily Value of Vitamin B6;
15% Daily Value of Vitamin E;
15% Daily Value of Manganese;
13% Daily Value of Vitamin A.

Pineapple - 1 cup includes these anti-inflammatories:

131% Daily Value of Vitamin C;
79% Daily Value of Manganese.

Salmon - 1 cup includes these anti-inflammatories:

236% Daily Value of Vitamin B12;
127% Daily Value of Vitamin D;
78.3% Daily Value of Selenium;
56.3% Daily Value of Vitamin B3;
55% Daily Value of Omega 3;
53.1% Daily Value of Protein;
52.1% Daily Value of Phosphorus;
37.6% Daily Value of Vitamin B6.

Bone Broth - Contains Chondroitin, Sulphates and Glucosamine which all help to reduce inflammation.

Coconut Oil - Contains antioxidants and compounds that have been shown to lower inflammation within the body.

Chapter #3 - General Benefits

****

This chapter is designed to give you some generalized benefits of Astaxanthin. To read up on some of the research articles for the various conditions it treats then please see section #2. However, if you are just looking for some general information, this section is for you.

Potent Antioxidant

As explained in Section #1, Astaxanthin is one of the most potent antioxidants you can take. If you would like to learn more about how antioxidants can benefit you, please check out Chapter #2.

Inflammation

Due to its anti-inflammatory properties, Astaxanthin has been shown to help with a variety of inflammatory conditions (i.e. Arthritis). However, unlike prescription medications, there are no risks of addiction or ulcers which come along with these medications.

Pain

Astaxanthin is a potent pain reliever, blocking the many different chemicals in your body which cause you to scream "Ouch".

Skin Health

Astaxanthin has been shown to help with skin moisture levels, as well as the smoothness/elasticity of the skin. On top of this, the antioxidant has been shown to help reduce wrinkles and help with spots/freckles.

Internal Sunscreen

Astaxanthin has powerful UV blocking properties which help to protect the fish from sun related damage. It has been shown to do the same for humans.

Energy

One of the most potent astaxanthin foods, sockeye salmon, has vibrant red flesh indicating its high levels of this antioxidant. It is now known that it is this level of astaxanthin which gives the salmon the energy to move upstream every year. It has been shown to also increase strength in humans and offer increased recovery from exercise.

Eye Health

As Astaxanthin can cross the retinal barrier, it has been shown to help diabetic retinopathy, macular degeneration and a whole host of other eye conditions.

Cortisol Reduction

Studies have shown that 8 weeks of Astaxanthin use can reduce cortisol levels by up to 23%. These high cortisol levels can contribute to increased blood glucose and fat levels, which are markers for diabetes and pre-diabetes.

****

SECTION 2 - RESEARCH

****

Chapter #4 - Allergies/Asthma

****

Allergy: When the immune system reacts to environmental factors that are harmless for most people, such as dust mites, pets, insects, mould, foods and some medicines and causes a histamine reaction.

Asthma: A respiratory condition that causes inflammation in the lungs, leading to spasms and difficulty breathing. Most often caused by an allergy or another form of hypersensitivity.

Types of Allergies

There are many different types of allergies that you may experience, such as:

- Cat Allergies;
- Dog Allergies;
- Egg Allergies;
- Gluten Allergies;
- Latex Allergies;
- Milk Allergies;
- Peanut Allergies;
- Pollen Allergies (Hay-fever);
- Shellfish Allergies.

Symptoms of Allergies

- Anaphylaxis - Rare but the most serious reaction;
- Sneezing, Itchy Runny Nose (Hay-fever);
- Itchy Red Rash (Hives);
- Itchy Red, Watery Eyes (Conjunctivitis);
- Abdominal Pain (Food Allergies);
- Wheezing, Chest Tightness, Shortness of Breath and Cough.

Symptoms of Asthma

- Coughing, especially at night or after intense exercise;
- Difficulty breathing;
- Chest tightness;
- Shortness of breath;
- Wheezing.

How Astaxanthin Can Help With Allergies

Astaxanthin is known to decrease inflammation as well as inhibit histamine production. On top of that, it has been shown to improve the effectiveness of pharmaceutical antihistamines.

Research (1) - "In Vitro Suppression of Lymphocyte activation in patients with seasonal allergic rhinitis and pollen-related asthma by cetrizine or azelastine in combination with ginkgolide B or Astaxanthin"

This study set out to determine if astaxanthin interacts with 2 different types of antihistamines to improve their ability to down regulate pathological immune activation. The results of this study demonstrated improvements in antihistamine effectiveness with the use of astaxanthin.

How Astaxanthin Can Help with Asthma

According to the study given, when astaxanthin is used in combination with ginkgo biloba and vitamin c, it is just as effective as ibuprofen at reducing inflammation associated with asthma.

Research (2) - "Summative Interaction between astaxanthin, ginkgo biloba extract and vitamin C in suppression of respiratory inflammation: a comparison with ibuprofen"

In this study, combinations of ginkgo biloba leaf extract, astaxanthin and vitamin C were evaluated for a summative dose effect in the inhibition of asthma-associated inflammation in asthmatic guinea pigs, in comparison to ibuprofen. Each parameter that was measured was significantly altered to a greater degree by drug combinations than by each drug independently.

The results found that the optimal combination was astaxanthin (10mg/kg), vitamin C (200mg/kg) and ginkgo biloba (10mg/kg). This combination resulted in counts of eosinophils and neutrophils (1.6 fold lower), macrophages (1.8 fold lower), cAMP (1.4 fold higher) and cGMP (2.04 fold higher) than in the non-asthmatic animals.

This study has shown that this combination is equal to or better in effectiveness than ibuprofen in relation to reducing inflammation associated with asthma.

Chapter #5 - Autoimmune Disorders

****

An Autoimmune condition is one whereby the immune system has gone crazy and has begun to attack healthy tissue. For instance, Autoimmune Hepatitis is when the immune system attacks the liver and Rheumatoid Arthritis is when it attacks the joints.

Types of Autoimmune Disorders

There are many different types of autoimmune disorders. Some will affect individual organs within the body, while others are systemic and affect the whole body.

Examples of Common Localized Autoimmune Conditions

> Autoimmune Hepatitis (Liver);
> Coeliac Disease (GI Tract);
> Diabetes - Type 1 (Pancreas);
> Hashimotos Thyroiditis (Thyroid); and
> Myasthenia Gravis (Nerves and Muscles).

Examples of Common Systemic Autoimmune Conditions

> Rheumatoid Arthritis;
> Sjogrens Syndrome; and
> Systemic Lupus Erythematosus (SLE).

Causes of Autoimmune Disorders

Autoimmune Disorders have a major genetic component to them, but even so, they still require a trigger to kickstart them.

Some of these triggers could include:

Environmental Pollution;
Nutritional Deficiencies;
Stress;
Toxins; or
Trauma.

How Astaxanthin Can Help With Autoimmunity

There are a couple of ways that Astaxanthin can help with Autoimmunity:

By Being A Potent Antioxidant

Oxidative stress plays a massive role in the development of autoimmune disease. Free radicals within the body begin to attack healthy cells, therefore causing these cells to lose their function and eventually destroying them.

By Being Potently Anti-Inflammatory

Inflammation is something that must be kept in check. Chronic inflammation is especially related to autoimmune conditions such as Rheumatoid Arthritis, Sjogrens Syndrome and Fibromyalgia.

Excessive levels of pro-inflammatory cytokines (such as those found in Rheumatoid Arthritis) are known to contribute towards the inflammatory syndrome that begins to destroy the joint cartilage, leading to these painful conditions.

Although not a lot of research has been done on the benefits of Astaxanthin on Autoimmune Disease, I have managed to find three research studies that demonstrate its potential benefits...

Recommended Dosage

Studies have shown that anywhere between 2 and 8mg per day is enough to boost immunity and reduce C Reactive Protein.

Research (3) - Autoimmune Hepatitis - Autoimmune Disorder of the Liver - "Protective effects of astaxanthin on ConA-induced autoimmune hepatitis by the JNK/p-JNK pathway-mediated inhibition of autophagy and apoptosis"

In this study, they set out to investigate the protective effects of astaxanthin on Con-A induced Autoimmune Hepatitis in mice.

They gave the mice astaxanthin supplementation daily at 2 different doses (20mg/kg and 40mg/kg). 14 days later, they induced autoimmune hepatitis in the mice.

The primary hepatocytes (liver cells) were pre-treated with astaxanthin for 24 hours before being stimulated with the pro-inflammatory cytokine TNF-a.

What they found was that astaxanthin did reduce the liver injury in the mice with autoimmune hepatitis.

Research (4) - Oral Lichen Planus - Autoimmune Disorder of the Oral Cavity - "Anti-Inflammatory effects of astaxanthin in the human gingival keratinocyte line NDUSD-1"

In this study they set out to evaluate whether astaxanthin is able to be used to improve Lichen Planus, by reducing inflammation caused by Escherichia Coli in human keratinocytes.

After the astaxanthin treatment, they found that the inflammatory cytokines decreased, and cell proliferation increased. This suggests that astaxanthin may be useful for improving chronic inflammation, such as that which is found in Oral Lichen Planus.

Research (5) - Sjogrens Syndrome - Autoimmune Disorder of the Salivary Glands and Tear Ducts - "Evaluation of therapeutic effects of astaxanthin on impairments in salivary secretion"

This study set out to examine the anti-oxidative capacity of Astaxanthin using a human salivary gland (HSY) epithelial cell line. They also performed a clinical study of Astaxanthin in 6 Sjogren patients and 6 normal individuals. In this study they quantified the volume of saliva secretion and the level of oxidative stress markers in the saliva. They found that Astaxanthin partially suppressed the hydrogen peroxide induced oxidation in the HSY cells and also increased the salivary output in both the Sjogren and Normal patients. The level of oxidative stress marker, hexanoyl-lysine in the saliva was reduced after Astaxanthin intake. Therefore, Astaxanthin may act as an ROS scavenger, providing benefit to Sjogren patients with impaired salivary secretion.

Chapter #6 - Benign Prostatic Hyperplasia

****

Also known as a benign (non-cancerous) enlargement or growth of the prostate gland. Although not life threatening, the symptoms can still create major issues with quality of life.

BPH is the most common prostate disease and it usually appears in men over the age of 40. Men with this disorder may not have symptoms straight away, but as time goes on, the symptoms may get worse.

Studies have shown that Astaxanthin, along with the herb Saw Palmetto is a powerful inhibitor of the 5-alpha reductase enzyme.

This enzyme is one responsible for converting testosterone to dihydrotestosterone (DHT) and by inhibiting it, both Astaxanthin and Saw Palmetto prevent the swelling of the prostate gland, and therefore also prevents the occurrence of Benign Prostatic Hyperplasia.

Symptoms of BPH

- Lower Urinary Tract Symptoms such as:
  - Hesitancy (taking longer than usual for the urine to evacuate);
  - Weak stream of urine;
  - Straining to urinate;
  - Dribbling after urination has finished;
  - Urinary retention;
  - Urgent feeling of needing to urinate;
  - A short time between needing to urinate;
  - A need to pass urine more than twice per night.
- Perineal Pain (Pain in the Perineum);
- Dysuria (Painful Urination);
- Haematuria (Blood in the Urine).

Causes of BPH

Although it isn't clear why the prostate enlarges, it is likely that it may be due to changes in the balance of sex hormones as the men get older.

Risk Factors for BPH

There are many factors that may increase the risk of a person suffering from BPH:

Aging

It is very rare for a man to suffer from BPH before the age of 40. About 1/3 of men experience symptoms by the age of 60 and about 1/2 by the age of 80.

Genetics

If you have a blood relative, such as a father or brother that has prostate issues, then it is more likely you will also have prostate problems.

Ethnicity

Prostate enlargement is more common in white and black men than in those of asian descent. However, black men may experience symptoms at a younger age than white men.

Diabetes/Heart Disease

It has been shown that the use of beta blockers and the occurrence of diabetes/heart disease may increase your risk of BPH.

Lifestyle Factors

Obesity may increase your risk of BPH, Exercise may decrease it.

Recommended Dosage

Studies have shown that anywhere between 4 and 8mg per day is sufficient for prostate health.

Research (6) - "A Preliminary investigation of the enzymatic inhibition of 5 alpha reduction and growth of prostatic carcinoma cell line LNCap-FGC by natural astaxanthin and saw palmetto in vitro"

In this study they set out to investigate the effect of astaxanthin and saw palmetto on the 5 alpha reductase enzyme inhibition as well as its impact on prostate cancer growth.

The results of this study show that astaxanthin demonstrates a 98% inhibition of 5 alpha reductase at 300mg/mL in vitro. The combination of the two showed a 20% greater inhibition of 5 alpha reductase than saw palmetto alone.

On top of this, it also showed that it decreased the growth of prostate cancer cells by 24% (at 0.1 mcg/mL) and 38% (at 0.01 mcg/mL). Saw Palmetto alone showed a 34% decrease (at 0.1 mcg/mL).

Chapter #7 - Blood Pressure

****

Blood Pressure is the pressure of the blood against the walls of the blood vessels. If the pressure is too high, it will put extra strain on your heart, possibly leading to heart attacks and strokes.

Your blood pressure will consist of 2 separate numbers. The top number is your systolic blood pressure and it is the pressure of your blood when your heart is beating.

The bottom number is your diastolic blood pressure and it is the pressure of the blood when your heart is at rest.

There are two main ways that Astaxanthin can help with Blood Pressure:

Reducing Oxidative Stress

Oxidative stress has been shown to be a major cause or contributor towards the development of blood pressure. Due to the fact that Astaxanthin is a potent antioxidant it also shows how it will help with the reduction of blood pressure.

Improving the Bio availability of Nitric Oxide

Nitric Oxide, also known as NO is your natural guard against hypertension. It has a powerful ability to regulate blood pressure by dilating your arteries.

One of the most interesting findings over the years regarding Nitric Oxide is that people with hypertension (amongst other disorders) seem to have impaired NO pathways.

Astaxanthin has been shown to increase the bio availability of nitric oxide in the body, therefore decreasing blood pressure.

Recommended Levels of Blood Pressure

Normal:	Less than 120/80
Prehypertension:	120-139/80-89
Stage 1 Hypertension:	140-159/90-99
Stage 2 Hypertension:	160+/100+
Over Age 60:	150+/90+

Risk Factors for Hypertension

Essential Hypertension (with no other associated conditions) is still a mysterious condition, but it has been linked to a number of risk factors:

- Family History;
- Greater incidence in men than women;
- Greater incidence in blacks than in whites, although this gap narrows around the age of 44;
- After the age of 65, black women have the greatest incidence of hypertension.

Causes of Hypertension

Although the actual cause of high blood pressure is not known, there are a number of factors that could increase the likelihood of it affecting you:

- Smoking;
- Obesity;
- Excessive Alcohol Consumption;
- Stress;
- Age;
- Genetics - Family History of Hypertension;
- Chronic Kidney Disease;
- Adrenal Disorders;
- Thyroid Disorders;
- Sleep Apnea;
- Being Too Sedentary.

Recommended Dosage

Studies have shown that 6mg of Astaxanthin per day is sufficient for lowering blood pressure levels.

Research (7) - "Astaxanthin reduces blood pressure and improves cardiovascular parameters in hypertensive rats"

In this study they set out to investigate the effects of an astaxanthin enriched diet on blood pressure and cardiac hypertrophy in hypertensive rats.

12-week old rats were treated for 8 weeks with a diet enriched with astaxanthin, at either 75mg/kg of body weight or 200mg/kg of body weight. The rats systolic blood pressure was monitored periodically throughout the study and they found that it was lower in those rats treated with astaxanthin than in the control grou

Research (8) - "High Dose Astaxanthin lowers blood pressure and increases insulin sensitivity in rats: are these effects interdependent?"

This study set out to examine the effects of astaxanthin at different doses on elevated blood pressure and glucose-insulin perturbations produced by heavy sucrose ingestion. They also examined the effects of Astaxanthin on blood pressure during restrained stress.

The rats were divided into 6 different groups, each group containing 8 rats. All the groups ate the same amount of sucrose, with the five test groups consisting of either captopril (30mg/kg), pioglitazone (15mg/kg), low astaxanthin (25mg/kg), medium astaxanthin (50mg/kg) and high astaxanthin (100mg/kg).

The study showed that at low doses of astaxanthin, systolic blood pressure was decreased with no change in insulin sensitivity. Increasing the dose of astaxanthin resulted in further lowering of systolic blood pressure, as well as increased insulin sensitivity. On top of that, astaxanthin at higher doses seemed to reduce the restrained stress in the rats and improve NO bio availability.

Chapter #8 - Brain Health

****

Within this chapter I will explain how Astaxanthin benefits the brain in general and then I will give you research studies showing how a number of neurological conditions are benefited with the use of Astaxanthin.

Astaxanthin is particularly beneficial in promoting brain health by preventing oxidative stress and reducing inflammation in the brain. Unlike many other antioxidants, it is able to cross the blood brain barrier effectively and therefore benefit the brain directly.

When chronic inflammation is present in the brain it can lead to numerous neurological conditions, such as:

- Parkinson's Disease;
- Huntington's Disease;
- Alzheimer's Disease;
- ALS (Lou Gehrig's Disease); and
- Dementia.

Astaxanthin has an amazing ability to reduce harmful free radicals known as peroxides by 50%. This is really important because people with Dementia and Alzheimers seem to have abnormal accumulation of these hydroperoxides in their red blood cells.

These effects are seen in as little as 12mg per day.

How Astaxanthin Can Help with Brain Health

There are a number of reasons why astaxanthin is beneficial for brain health:

- As mentioned above, it crosses the blood brain barrier, therefore directly affecting the brain.
- It helps with the reduction of blood pressure, therefore may minimize the risk of stroke;
- May improve memory in Dementia;
- May boost intelligence and memory; and
- May help prevent brain damage due to Ischemia.

Recommended Dosage

As mentioned above, 12mg per day is a great dosage for reducing oxidation and free radicals in the brain.

Research (9) - "Astaxanthin improves behavioral disorder and oxidative stress in prenatal valproic acid induced mice model of Autism."

In this study they administered Valproic Acid intraperitoneally into the pregnant mice on day 12.5 of the pregnancy. On day 25, these Valproic exposed groups were split in two (one was the control and one was the treatment group).

The treatment group was given 2mg/kg of Astaxanthin for a total of 4 weeks. A number of tests were carried out on the mice on day 26 so as to confirm that they did exhibit signs of autism. When these tests were done, they displayed delayed eye opening, longer time to respond to pain, poor sociability, high level of anxiety and an increased level of oxidative stress.

Treatment with the astaxanthin was shown to improve the behavioral disorder and reduce the oxidative stress in the brain and the liver.

Research (10) - "Astaxanthin supplementation enhances adult hippocampal neurogenesis and spatial memory in mice"

This study set out to determine the effect of Astaxanthin on adult hippocampal neurogenesis and spatial memory in mice.

To do this, they fed mice an astaxanthin supplemented diet and then assessed the adult hippocampal neurogenesis as well as the hippocampus dependent cognitive function.

Results reveal that astaxanthin enhanced cell proliferation and survival at 0.1% and 0.5% dosages. Therefore, it was shown to enhance AHN and spatial memory.

Research (11) - "Impact of astaxanthin enriched algal powder of Haematococcus pluvialis on memory improvement in BALB/c mice"

In this study they set out to determine the impact of astaxanthin enriched algal powder on auxiliary memory improvement in BALB/c mice for 30 days.

Over a couple of weeks these mice were put through a series of tests to determine their latency, distance, speed and the directions they take to the platforms. What they found in this study was that a middle dosage of H Pluvialis meals (1.3mg astaxanthin/kg body weight) shortened the latency and distance required for the mice to find the hidden platform.

Mice supplemented with the algal meal hesitantly turned around the original hidden platform, but the placebo mice easily forgot the original location and accepted the visible platform as a safe place.

These results indicate that mice supplemented with astaxanthin has the auxiliary property of memory improvement. When looking at dosages, they found that mice supplemented with low amounts of astaxanthin is more beneficial in improving the memory than higher amounts.

Research (12) - *"Astaxanthin reduces ischemic brain injury in adult rats"*

This study set out to examine whether astaxanthin can protect against ischemic injury in the mammalian brain. Adult rats were injected with astaxanthin or placebo prior to a 60 min cerebral artery occlusion (MCAo).

Astaxanthin was still present in the infarction area at 70-75 minutes after onset of MCAo.

Results showed that treatment with astaxanthin, as opposed to placebo increased locomotor activity in stroke rats and reduced cerebral infarction.

The data in this study suggests that astaxanthin can reduce ischemia related brain injury in brain tissue by inhibiting oxidative stress, glutamate release and anti-apoptosis.

Chapter #9 - Cancer

****

There have been numerous animal studies which have shown that Astaxanthin is useful when preventing and/or treating cancer. These research articles have shown benefits in treating Breast Cancer, Colon Cancer, and Leukemia, to name a few.

How Astaxanthin can help with Cancer

1. Astaxanthin has been shown to inhibit cell cancer growth in Breast Cancer, Leukemia and possibly a variety of other cancers.
2. Astaxanthin decreases lipid peroxidation in both Breast Cancer and Colon Cancer.
3. Beta Carotene, Astaxanthin and Canthaxanthin have all been shown to decrease the number of mammary tumors.

There are many ways that astaxanthin may help to protect against cancer, including:

- By limiting free radical production in the oxidatively stressed tissues, therefore reducing the DNA damage which initiates various cancers.
- By reducing inflammatory mediators that allow pre-cancerous cells to develop into full grown tumors.
- By improving the health of the cells, therefore improving the body's resistance to cancer.
- By upregulating PPARγ and P21 and downregulates cyclin D1 in a dose dependent manner. PPARγ plays an inhibitory role in cancer cell proliferation and growth.

Recommended Dosage

For the treatment of cancer, between 4mg and 12mg per day has been found to be beneficial.

Research (13) Breast Cancer - "A comparison of the anticancer activities of dietary beta-carotene, canthaxanthin and astaxanthin in mice in vivo"

This study set out to compare the growth of mammary tumours across three separate antioxidants - beta carotene, astaxanthin and canthaxanthin.

They took 8-week old female BALB/c mice and fed them diets consisting of each of these antioxidants.

After the mice had been on the diet for three weeks they inoculated them with breast tumours. No carotenoids were present in the plasma or tumour tissues of the un-supplemented mice.

They found that all three carotenoids decreased the volume of mammary tumours, but the growth of the tumours was inhibited significantly more in those fed astaxanthin, as was the lipid peroxidation (free radical) activity in the tumours.

Research (14) Colon Cancer - "Antioxidative and antiproliferative effects of astaxanthin during the initiation stages of 1,2-dimethyl hydrazine-induced experimental colon carcinogenesis"

In this rat study, they set out to determine the chemo-preventive effect of astaxanthin on lipid peroxidation, antioxidant status, total number of aberrant crypt foci and cell proliferation.

These rats were administered DMH induced colon cancer twice a week for 2 weeks.

Astaxanthin was administered before and after the induction. After the end of 16 weeks they found that pre-treatment with astaxanthin markedly reduced the degree of histological lesions, ACF development and lowered lipid peroxidation.

Research (15) Leukemia - "Carotenoids inhibit proliferation and regulate expression of peroxisome proliferators-activated receptor gamma (PPARγ) in K562 cancer cells"

In this study they set out to determine what role PPARγ had on the inhibition of leukemia K562 cells.

The results of this study determined that beta carotene, astaxanthin, capsanthin and bixin all inhibited the proliferation and decreased the viability of leukemia K562 cells in both dose and time dependent manners.

They also induced cell apoptosis and interfered with cell cycle progression.

Chapter #10 - Cardiovascular Disease (Atherosclerosis)

****

Build-up of fats, cholesterol and other factors in and on your artery walls, which can restrict your blood flow.

Because of Astaxanthins potent anti-inflammatory and anti-oxidative properties, natural astaxanthin is a great tonic for the heart. It has many properties which can help people prevent heart disease and minimize the risk of heart attack and stroke.

Symptoms

What symptoms you experience in response to atherosclerosis will depend on what arteries are affected:

- Heart - Chest Pain or Pressure.
- Brain - Sudden numbness or weakness in arms or legs, Difficult or Slurred Speech, Loss of Vision in one eye, Drooping muscles in your face.
- Arms or Legs - Leg pain when walking.
- Kidneys - High Blood Pressure or Kidney Failure.

Causes

- High Blood Pressure;
- High Cholesterol;
- High Triglycerides;
- Smoking;
- Insulin Resistance, Obesity or Diabetes;
- Excessive Inflammation.

Recommended Dosage

For high cholesterol and heart health, 6, 12 and 18mg per day has been taken.

How Astaxanthin can help with Cardiovascular Disease

- Increases HDL (Good) Cholesterol;
- Reduce LDL Cholesterol;
- Reduces Triglyceride Levels;
- Prevents Lipid Oxidation;
- Lowering Blood Pressure.

Research (16) - "Effect of an oral astaxanthin prodrug (CDX-085) on lipoprotein levels and progression of atherosclerosis in LDL-R (-/-) and ApoE (-/-) mice"

In this study, they set out to analyse whether delivery of astaxanthin reduces plasma lipoprotein levels and the progression of atherosclerosis in low density lipoprotein receptor negative and apolipoprotein E deficient mice.

3 mouse studies were conducted:

* 1 - 16 wild type and 16 LDL-R mice on 0.5% cholesterol diet supplemented with 0.0%, 0.08%, 0.2% and 0.4% astaxanthin for 4 weeks.

* 2 - 36 male LDL-R mice were randomized to a 0.5% cholesterol chow diet or 0.5% cholesterol chow fortified with .08% or 0.5% cholesterol chow with 0.4% astaxanthin for 12 weeks.

* 3 - 34 male ApoE mice were randomized in the same fashion as study #2 and fed similar diets for 9 weeks.

They found that the astaxanthin prodrug CDX-085 is distributed among lipoproteins to lower total cholesterol and atherosclerosis in LDL-R mice and reduce triglyceride levels in ApoE mice.

Chapter #11 - Diabetes/Insulin Resistance

****

Insulin Resistance - A state or condition where your body has a lowered level response to insulin.

Type 2 Diabetes - When the Beta Cells of the pancreas produce insulin but can't use it effectively because of its resistance to insulin.

Type 1 Diabetes - Also known as juvenile diabetes or insulin dependent diabetes, it is a chronic condition where the pancreas produces little or no insulin.

Symptoms

Insulin Resistance

- Weight Gain around the middle;
- Lethargy;
- Hunger;
- Difficulty Concentrating;
- High Blood Pressure/High Glucose Levels.

Diabetes

- Extreme thirst or hunger;
- Feeling hungry even after a meal;
- Frequent or increased urination;
- Tingling sensations in your hands and feet;
- Feeling more tired than usual.

Causes

- High Carbohydrate Diet;
- Poor quality diet; and
- Sedentary Lifestyle.

How Astaxanthin can help with Diabetes/Diabetic Complications and Insulin Resistance

- Enhances GLUT-4 translocation and glucose uptake, therefore improving insulin resistance.

- Acts as a potent antioxidant, therefore protecting the cells from oxidative stress and improving insulin resistance (17).

- Improves the health of the islet cells in the pancreas and helps to decrease the glucose toxicity associated with diabetes.

- May protect against diabetic nephropathy through the ROS scavenging effect in the mitochondria of the mesangial cells (44).

- It has been shown to have neuroprotective effects and reduce ocular oxidative stress and inflammation (45).

- It activates the PI3K/Akt pathway and attenuates oxidative stress, reducing Type 2 Diabetic Associated Cognitive Decline (46).

- It provides neuroprotection against diabetes-induced sickness behaviour by inhibiting inflammation and activating CBS expression in the brain (47).

Recommended Dosage

2mg per day is enough to help reverse insulin resistance and protect against progressing to Diabetes.

Research (17) - "Impact of divergent effects of astaxanthin on insulin signaling in L6 cells"

This study explored the effect of astaxanthin on insulin signalling and investigated whether it improves cytokine and free fatty acid induced insulin resistance in vitro.

It examined the effect of astaxanthin on insulin stimulated glucose transporter 4 (GLUT-4) translocation, glucose uptake and insulin signalling in cultured rat L6 muscle cells.

They observed that astaxanthin improved insulin resistance associated with diabetes by enhancing the GLUT-4 translocation and glucose uptake and reducing oxidative stress.

These results indicate that astaxanthin is a very effective antioxidant for ameliorating insulin resistance by protecting cells from oxidative stress generated by various stimuli such as TNFa and Palmitate.

Research (18) - "Astaxanthin prevents loss of insulin signalling and improves glucose metabolism in liver of insulin resistant"

This study investigated the effects of astaxanthin on insulin signalling and glucose metabolism in the liver of mice fed a high fat and a high fructose diet.

To do this, adult male mice were fed a normal chow or high fat high fructose diet. After 15 days, mice in each group were split into 2 smaller groups and given 2mg/kg Astaxanthin in olive oil for 45 days.

At the end of the 60 days, the mice not fed astaxanthin were insulin resistant but the mice that were fed astaxanthin showed a marked improvement in insulin sensitivity parameters.

Research (19) - *"Astaxanthin protects beta-cells against glucose toxicity in diabetic db/db mice"*

The aim of this study was to examine whether astaxanthin can have a beneficial effect on the progressive destruction of pancreatic beta cells in mice.

For this study, they used diabetic C57Bl mice and then a control group. At 6 weeks of age, Astaxanthin treatment was started and its effects were evaluated at 10,14 and 18 weeks of age by taking non-fasting blood glucose levels, glucose tolerance test and beta cell histology.

The non-fasting blood glucose level was higher in the diabetic mice than the control group but the higher level of blood glucose in these diabetic mice was significantly decreased after treatment with astaxanthin.

Also, the ability of the islet cells in the pancreas to secrete insulin was preserved in the group taking astaxanthin. Therefore, this shows that astaxanthin may be beneficial for reducing glucose toxicity.

Chapter #12 - Dyspepsia

****

Also known as indigestion, it is a condition characterized by upper abdominal symptoms which can cause extreme distress in the individual.

Dyspepsia is an incredibly common condition which affects about 1/4 of the adult population. It is most commonly connected with the Helicobacter Pylori bacteria.

This H Pylori infection increases the oxidative stress in the stomach lining, which shows why astaxanthin can be useful in treating this condition.

Symptoms of Dyspepsia (Indigestion)

- Pain or Discomfort;
- Bloating;
- Feeling of fullness with very little intake of food;
- Feeling of unusual fullness following meals;
- Nausea;
- Loss of Appetite;
- Heartburn;
- Regurgitation of food or acid;
- Belching.

Causes of Dyspepsia

- Burped up stomach juices and gases caused by GERD or Hiatal Hernia;
- Irritable Bowel Syndrome;
- Peptic Ulcer/Duodenal Ulcers;
- Lactose Intolerance;
- Gallbladder Pain or Inflammation;
- Anxiety/Depression;
- Caffeine/Alcohol;

- Certain Medications, such as aspirin, antibiotics, steroids, digoxin and theophylline;
- Stomach Cancer.

How Astaxanthin Can Help with Dyspepsia

Anti-Inflammatory Properties

As mentioned above, Dyspepsia is often caused by the bacteria H Pylori which causes a great amount of inflammation in the gut. Because of its anti-inflammatory properties, astaxanthin can reduce this gut inflammation.

Inhibits H Pylori Growth

As seen in the studies below, Astaxanthin has been shown to inhibit the growth of H Pylori, as well as reduce the immune response triggered by the bacteria.

Upregulates CD4 Lymphocytes and Downregulates CD8 Lymphocytes

CD4 Lymphocytes are known as the helper cells and are responsible for leading the attack against infections (i.e. H Pylori). CD8 on the other hand is also known as killer cells and are responsible for ending the immune response. Astaxanthin modulates this immune response.

Recommended Dosage

If you are wanting to treat Dyspepsia, as much as 40mg per day, in 3-4 divided doses, over a period of 4 weeks has been found to be effective.

Research (20) - "Treatment of H Pylori infected mice with antioxidant astaxanthin reduces gastric inflammation, bacterial load and modulates cytokine release by splenocytes"

In this study they set out to investigate whether dietary antioxidant induced modulation of H Pylori in mice affected the cytokines produced by H Pylori specific T Cells (Immune Cells).

Results showed that treating these H Pylori infected mice with the algal extract (astaxanthin) reduces bacterial load and gastric inflammation.

Research (21) - "Gastric Inflammatory Markers and Interleukins in Patients with Functional Dyspepsia treated with Astaxanthin"

In this study they set out to investigate the effect of astaxanthin on gastric inflammation in patients with functional dyspepsia.

44 patients were included (21 taking 40mg of astaxanthin daily and 23 taking placebo).

They found a significant decrease in gastric inflammation in both groups and although there was not a significant change in the density of H Pylori during or after treatment, there was a significant upregulation of CD4 and downregulation of CD8 in the patients with H Pylori patients treated with astaxanthin.

Chapter #13 - Eye Health

****

Unlike many of the other antioxidants, Astaxanthin is able to cross the blood-retinal barrier to the eyes. By crossing this barrier, it is able to accumulate within the retina and protect against free radicals.

Astaxanthin is then able to help the tissues vascular health and improve vision, reduce irritation and blurry eyes and prevent eyestrain/eye fatigue.

Tso, alongside other researchers (and research articles included below) have shown that Astaxanthin is able to prevent light induced damage as well as damage to the inner retinal layers.

Because of this, Astaxanthin has been shown to be beneficial in treating a whole host of eye disorders, such as:

- Eyestrain;
- Age Related Macular Degeneration;
- Diabetic Neuropathy;
- Venous Occlusion;
- Glaucoma;
- Cataracts; and
- Inflammatory Eye Disease.

How Astaxanthin Can Help With Eye Health

1. Because Astaxanthin is able to cross the blood-retinal barrier and therefore works on the oxidation of the retina directly;
2. Helps vascular health within the eyes;
3. Can ameliorate or prevent light induced damage, photoreceptor cell damage, ganglion cell damage and damage to the neurons of the inner retinal layers.

Recommended Dosage

Studies have shown that a dose of 6mg Astaxanthin per day is sufficient for eye health.

Research (22) - "Eyestrain - Effects of Astaxanthin on Eyestrain Induced By Accommodative Dysfunction"

This study set out to determine the supplementation of effects of astaxanthin on subjects suffering from visual display terminal induced visual fatigue.

They divided the subjects into two groups. Placebo and then a group taking 6mg Astaxanthin per day. They were kept on this regime for 4 weeks and then the groups visual accommodation was evaluated, and a questionnaire was done to evaluate eye fatigue.

They found that 6mg of astaxanthin per day from an algal extract can improve the eye fatigue. They also showed that astaxanthin can be safely consumed at this level as recommended by healthy doctors.

Research (23) - "Retinal Capillary Blood Flow - The Effect of Astaxanthin on Retinal Capillary Blood Flow in Normal Volunteers"

This study set out to determine the effect of astaxanthin on retinal capillary blood flow in normal volunteers. It consisted of 36 volunteers who were split into 2 groups. One group consisted of 18 subjects who received 6mg/day of Astaxanthin for 4 weeks and the other group consisted of 18 subjects receiving a placebo.

Changes in blood pressure, blood cell counts, fasting plasma glucose level, fasting plasma astaxanthin level, retinal capillary blood flow, intraocular pressure and level of eye strain were all measured before and after the supplementation.

After 4 weeks of supplementation, they found that the retinal capillary blood flow was significantly higher in the astaxanthin group, while the placebo group had not changed at all.

Research (24) Cataracts - "Effect of astaxanthin on cataract formation induced by glucocorticoids in the chick embryo"

This study set out to determine whether astaxanthin prevents cataract formation induced by glucocorticoids in the chick embryo.

They found that administration of astaxanthin into the embryos decreased the lens opacity dose dependently and higher levels of astaxanthin prevented loss of reduced glutathione from the lens.

This suggests that astaxanthin protects glucocorticoid induced cataracts in chick embryos.

Chapter #14 - Fitness

****

We all know that exercise is an important part of everyday life. It is critical for maintaining optimal health, but how much we should do is still under discussion.

Exercise is not something that goes by the adage "more is better" because excessive exercise actually creates more free radicals and therefore requires extra antioxidants and anti-inflammatory nutrients to offset this oxidation.

As you can see from the studies below, if you are struggling with recovering from your workouts, then astaxanthin may be just what you need.

After compiling the information from all of these studies, it shows some serious promise in helping you with your exercise and your recovery period.

How Astaxanthin Can Help with Fitness and Recovery

- Causes an increased utilization of fatty acids as an energy source, therefore allowing you to burn fat for fuel instead of glucose. Great for those on a ketogenic diet.
- It decreases lactic acid build-up, therefore improving recovery time.
- It can prevent exercise induced free radical build-up.
- Has been found to significantly increase power output and time trial results.

Recommended Dosage

For exercise capacity, it is recommended for you to take 8mg of astaxanthin prior to exercise and 8mg afterwards.

Research (25) - "Effects of Astaxanthin Supplementation on Exercise Induced Fatigue in Mice"

In this study they set out to determine the effect of astaxanthin on endurance capacity in male mice aged 4 weeks. For 5 weeks they were given either vehicle or astaxanthin (1.2, 6 or 30 mg/kg).

The results indicated the following:
* The astaxanthin group showed a significant increase in swimming time to exhaustion compared to the control group.
* Blood lactate concentration in the astaxanthin group was significantly lower than in the control group.
* In the astaxanthin group, non-esterified fatty acids (NEFA) and plasma glucose were significantly higher than the control group after swimming.
* Astaxanthin significantly decreased fat accumulation.

These results indicate that the astaxanthin causes an improvement in swimming endurance because of its increased utilization of fatty acids as an energy source.

Research (26) - "The astaxanthin-induced improvement in lipid metabolism during exercise is mediated by a PGC-1a increase in skeletal muscle"

This study investigated the effect of astaxanthin intake on lipid metabolism associated with aerobic exercise.

The mice were split into 4 groups - Sedentary, Sedentary with Astaxanthin, Exercise and Exercise with Astaxanthin. After 2 weeks of treatment, the exercise groups performed treadmill running at 25 meters/minute for 30 minutes. Immediately after the running, intermuscular pH was measured, and blood was collected for measurements.

The results of the study showed that levels of plasma fatty acids were significantly decreased in the exercised astaxanthin treated mice, compared to those fed a normal diet. It also found that the intermuscular pH was decreased with exercise (more lactic acid buildup), and this decrease was inhibited by astaxanthin. PGC-1α was elevated in skeletal muscle in the astaxanthin treated group, which can lead to acceleration of lipid utilization through activation of mitochondrial aerobic metabolism.

Research (27) - "Effect of Astaxanthin Supplementation on Muscle Damage and Oxidative Stress markers in elite young soccer players"

This study examined the effect of astaxanthin supplementation on muscle enzymes as indirect markers of muscle damage, oxidative stress markers and antioxidant response in elite young soccer players.

In this study they took 32 male elite soccer players who were randomly assigned in a double-blind fashion to either the astaxanthin or a placebo group. 90 days of supplementation, the athletes were required to perform a 2- hour bout of acute exercise.

Before and after 90 days of supplementation, blood samples were taken, and the following markers were tested:

* Thiobarbituric Acid Reacting Substances (TBARS);

* Advanced Oxidation Protein Products (AOPP);

* Superoxide Anion (o2);

* Total Antioxidative Status (TAS);

* Sulphydril Groups (SH);

* Superoxide Dismutase (SOD);

* Serum Creatine Kinase (CK); and

* Aspartate Aminotransferase (AST).

The results of the study showed that soccer training and soccer exercise were associated with excessive production of free radicals and oxidative stress, which diminishes the antioxidant system efficiency.

Astaxanthin supplementation can prevent exercise induced free radical production and depletion of non-enzymatic antioxidant defence in young soccer players.

Research (28) - "Effect of Astaxanthin on cycling time trial performance"

The researchers in this study set out to examine the effect of astaxanthin on metabolism and cycling time trial performance.

To do this, they randomly assigned 21 competitive cyclists to 28 days of encapsulated astaxanthin (4mg/day) or placebo. They made them complete a VO2 Max test and then a 2-hour pre-exhaustion ride on a separate day, after a 10 hour fast.

Overall, they observed significant improvements in the 20km time trial in the astaxanthin group but not the placebo group. The astaxanthin group also significantly increased power output, compared to the placebo group.

Research (29) - "Astaxanthin limits exercise induced skeletal and cardiac muscle damage in mice"

In this study they investigated the effect of astaxanthin supplementation on the oxidative damage induced by strenuous exercise in mouse skeletal muscle and heart.

7-week old mice were divided into 3 groups - rested control, intense exercise and exercise with astaxanthin. After 3 weeks of exercise acclimation, both of the exercise groups ran on a treadmill at 28 meters/minute until exhaustion.

Astaxanthin decreased the level of various pro-oxidants and attenuated exercise-induced damage in skeletal muscle and heart, including an associated infiltration that induces further damage.

Chapter #15 - Kidney Disease

****

Gradual loss of kidney function.

The kidneys are responsible for removing waste products and excess fluid from the body. They are also responsible for the critical regulation of the body's salt, potassium and acid content, as well as the production of hormones and vitamins that affect the function of other organs.

Types of Kidney Disease

- **Hereditary Disorders** - Generally produce clinical symptoms from teenage years to adulthood. The most common one is polycystic kidney disease.
- **Congenital Disease** - Involves malformation of genitourinary tract and usually leads to obstruction which produces infection and/or destruction of kidney tissue.
- **Acquired Kidney Disease** - These are numerous but the most common one is glomerulonephritis.
- **Kidney Stones** - Very common. The pain can be extremely severe in the side and back.

Symptoms of Kidney Disease

- Burning or difficulty urinating;
- Increase in the frequency of urination;
- Passage of blood in the urine;
- Puffiness around the eyes, swelling of the hands and feet;
- Pain in the small of the back just below the ribs;
- High blood pressure.

How Astaxanthin can help with Kidney Disease

The main reason that astaxanthin is able to help with kidney disease is because of its antioxidant ability. In studies, they found that astaxanthin preserves kidney function, reduces cell death, reduces inflammation and reduces oxidation.

Recommended Dosage

For Renal patients it is recommended to take 12mg of astaxanthin for a period of one year, split into 3 doses.

Research (30) - "Effect of Astaxanthin on kidney function impairment and oxidative stress induced by mercuric chloride in rats"

This study set out to evaluate the ability of astaxanthin to prevent HgCl Nephrotoxicity.

To do this, rats were injected with HgCl, 6 hours after astaxanthin had been administered and were killed 12 hours after HgCl exposure.

The results showed that astaxanthin could have a beneficial role against HgCl toxicity by preventing lipid and protein oxidation, changes in the activity of antioxidant enzymes and histopathological changes.

Research (31) - "Astaxanthin attenuates early acute kidney injury following severe burns in rats by ameliorating oxidative stress and mitochondrial related apoptosis"

This study attempted to explore the potential protection of astaxanthin against early post burn acute kidney injury and its possible mechanisms of action.

After astaxanthin treatment, renal tubular injury and the levels of serum creatinine and neutrophil gelatinase-associated lipocalin were improved.

The data from this study suggested that astaxanthin does protect against early acute kidney injury following severe burns in rats.

Chapter #16 – Non-Alcoholic Fatty Liver Disease

****

The accumulation of fat in the liver of people who drink little or no alcohol.

Non-alcoholic fatty liver disease is an incredibly common condition which often comes with very little signs or symptoms. However, for many, this condition can cause fat around the liver which causes inflammation and scarring.

Types of Fatty Liver Disease

- **Non-alcoholic Fatty Liver** - Not life threatening but can cause unnecessary fat around the liver.
- **Non-alcoholic Steatohepatitis** - A little more serious than non-alcoholic fatty liver. This is where the fat causes inflammation in the liver and it can lead to scarring of the liver (cirrhosis).
- **Non-alcoholic fatty liver disease associated cirrhosis** - This is when scarring gets so bad it can lead to liver failure.

Symptoms

Normally it is very rare to see any signs or symptoms for this condition. However, if it is severe you may experience:

- Fatigue;
- Pain in the Upper Right Abdomen; and
- Weight Loss.

Risk Factors

- High Cholesterol Levels;
- High Triglyceride Levels;
- Metabolic Syndrome;

- Obesity;
- Polycystic Ovarian Syndrome;
- Type 2 Diabetes;
- Hypothyroidism;
- Hyperthyroidism.

Recommended Dosage

As insulin resistance and fatty liver often go hand in hand, 2mg of astaxanthin per day should be sufficient.

How Astaxanthin can help with Non-Alcoholic Fatty Liver Disease

Astaxanthin is very effective at improving hepatic inflammation and fibrosis, as well as inhibition of lipid peroxidation (oxidation of lipids).

Research (32) - "Non-Alcoholic Fatty Liver Disease - Astaxanthin prevents and reverses diet-induced insulin resistance and steatohepatitis in mice: A comparison with Vitamin E"

In this study they set out to compare the effectiveness of Vitamin E to that of Astaxanthin when it came to treating steatohepatitis/fatty liver disease.

The results from this study concluded that:

Astaxanthin inhibited lipid peroxidation more potently than Vitamin E. Astaxanthin also improved hepatic inflammation and fibrosis by increasing the M1 type Macrophages/Kupffer cells and Stellate cells.

Therefore, they found astaxanthin was more effective at preventing and treating fatty liver disease than Vitamin E and may be a novel and promising treatment for this condition.

Chapter #17 - Pain

****

An uncomfortable, unpleasant sensation associated with actual or potential tissue damage. Pain is not a condition but is more a symptom.

Due to the potent anti-inflammatory properties of astaxanthin, it stands to reason that it is also effective against a host of chronic conditions which cause extreme pain.

Studies have shown that astaxanthin is not only useful against joint inflammation (i.e. Rheumatoid arthritis), but it also reduces nuclear kappa beta which is the master switch for the inflammatory response.

Tumor Necrosis Factor and other pro inflammatory cytokines have also been shown to be reduced with the use of astaxanthin.

Other Supplements for Pain

- **MSM** - This supplement has been shown to soften scar tissue, improve blood supply to the affected area, reduce muscle spasms and modulate inflammation. To read up more about this supplement, check out my book "MSM Uncovered";

- **Proteolytic Enzymes** - These have been shown to reduce C-Reactive Protein, Arterial Plaques, Blood Clots and Scar Tissue.

- **Turmeric, Ginger and Boswellia** - These are all anti-inflammatory herbs that have been found to be extremely beneficial in reducing pain, swelling and inflammation, when taken in very large doses.

- **Probiotics** - As chronic pain is often a sign of a leaky gut or infections in the gut, then probiotics will help to neutralize the toxins caused by the bad bacteria in the gut and fight back.

- **Magnesium** - This supplement is very important for relaxing muscles, maximising blood flow and allowing various nutrients to be delivered into the cells. To read up more about this supplement, check out my book "Magnificent Magnesium".

Recommended Dosage

Studies have shown that as little as 4mg per day is sufficient to improve the pain score of people with rheumatoid arthritis. Therefore, large doses are not required to be of benefit. Some even say it is as effective as their prescription medications.

Research (33) - "Effects of Astaxanthin from Litopenaeus Vannamei on Carrageenan-Induced Oedema and Pain Behaviour in Mice"

In this study they investigated whether astaxanthin can reduce the pain and inflammation associated with carrageenan induction in mouse paws. The study showed interesting effects from the astaxanthin treatment. It showed an inhibition of paw oedema, an increase in pain threshold and a decrease in the inflammation markers. * They found the effect was comparable to the common anti-inflammatory Indomethacin, however because of the cardiovascular and GI symptoms of this drug, astaxanthin may be a great alternative.

Chapter #18 - Peptic Ulcers

****

Classified as an open sore that is located in the lining of the stomach, oesophagus or upper small intestine. Gastric Ulcers are those that occur in the stomach. Duodenal Ulcers are those that occur in the upper portion of the small intestine.

About 4% of the population suffers from a peptic ulcer of some sort, with about 10% of the population developing an ulcer at some point in their life.

Symptoms of a Peptic Ulcer

- Abdominal Pain - Especially around meal times. With Duodenal Ulcers the pain appears about 3 hours after eating;
- Bloating;
- Abdominal Fullness;
- Nausea and Vomiting;
- Loss of Appetite;
- Weight Loss;
- Vomiting of Blood; or
- Gastric or Duodenal Perforation (very rare).

Cause of Peptic Ulcers

There are two main causes of Peptic Ulcers:

H Pylori

Chronic inflammation due to Helicobacter Pylori is a major causative factor. As mentioned in the section on "Dyspepsia", Astaxanthin is able to reduce the growth of H Pylori.

NSAID's

Chronic use of anti-inflammatory medications can lead to gastric ulcers. The gastric mucosa is essential for protecting itself from gastric acid with a special layer of mucus. This requires prostaglandins to help form this mucosa.

Unfortunately, NSAID's will stop the production of these prostaglandins, therefore causing burning from the stomach acid and leading to peptic ulcers.

How Astaxanthin Can Help with Peptic Ulcers

Reducing Incidence and Growth of H Pylori

To learn more about how Astaxanthin protects against H Pylori, please read the section on Dyspepsia.

By Raising Antioxidant Enzyme Levels In The Stomach

Astaxanthin ester pre-treatment has been shown to significantly raise antioxidant enzyme levels such as superoxide dismutase, catalase and glutathione perioxidase, therefore protecting against the injury of gastric mucin (a large glycoprotein which protects the stomach from acid, pathogens and trauma).

Recommended Dosage

As with Dyspepsia, up to 40mg per day can be useful in treating stomach issues. Start at a lower dose and move up until you reach optimal benefits.

Research (34) - "Protective effects of astaxanthin from Paracoccus Carotinifaciens on murine gastric ulcer models"

In this study they set out to investigate the effect of astaxanthin on gastric mucosal damage in the gastric ulcer models. The mice were pre-treated with astaxanthin 1 hour before ulcer induction.

The results indicated that astaxanthin decreased the extent of HCL/ethanol and acidified aspirin induced gastric ulcers. It was also found to have free radical scavenging activities against various free radical markers.

This suggests that astaxanthin has antioxidant properties and exerts a protective effect against ulcer formation.

Research (35) – "Therapeutic effect of astaxanthin on acetic acid induced gastric ulcer in rats"

In this study they investigated the therapeutic effect of astaxanthin on acetic acid-induced gastric ulcer in rats. These rats were divided into a control group, an ulcer control group and 3 astaxanthin groups (5mg/kg, 10mg/kg and 25mg/kg).

After administering the astaxanthin for 10 consecutive days, all the rats were culled and the area of the ulcer plus the levels of various markers were measured.

Compared with the ulcer control group, the astaxanthin groups all showed a decreased area of ulceration. This showed that astaxanthin has good therapeutic effects on acetic acid-induced gastric ulcer in rats.

Chapter #19 - Skin Health

****

Astaxanthin has been shown to be exceptionally beneficial when it comes to skin health and repair. In fact, actress Gwyneth Paltrow and supermodel Heidi Klum both use astaxanthin to help their skin.

Skin Care Benefits

- Fights Wrinkles;
- Improves Skin Elasticity;
- Reduces visible signs of UV aging within four to six weeks of use;
- Maintains a youthful appearance;
- Reverses premature signs of ageing;
- Reduces the risk of skin cancer.

What Type of Astaxanthin should be taken for the skin?

When ingested, astaxanthin is distributed throughout the whole body, but only a small amount of it ends up in the skin. However, topical astaxanthin is well absorbed when used in a cream or lotion.

Remember when using topical astaxanthin though that it may give a slight tint to your skin (not bad if you are looking for a tan). You are able to find topicals online. See my section on "How Do I Find It" at the back of this book to find out how.

How Astaxanthin can benefit the Skin

- It blocks a modest amount of UV light directly;

- Neutralizes some of the free radicals induced by UV radiation and responsible for some of the sun damage;

- Appears to inhibit the induction of matrix metalloproteinases (MMP) by UV light;

- It has an ability to regulate so call gap junctions, which are channels of cell to cell communication that is common in skin cells such as fibroblasts.

- Regulates the expression of inflammatory cytokines, therefore decreasing the scratching and intensity of *Atopic Dermatitis.*

- Exhibits anti-allergic and anti-inflammatory effects associated with *Contact Dermatitis.*

Recommended Dosage

For optimal skin health, 2mg of astaxanthin is recommended, twice a day, with breakfast and dinner.

Research (36) - "Cosmetic Benefits of Astaxanthin on human subjects"

This study set out to determine if astaxanthin was able to improve wrinkles, age spots, skin texture and moisture content of the skin. In this study, they took 30 healthy female subjects for 8 weeks and had them combine 6mg per day of oral supplementation mixed with 2ml per day of topical astaxanthin.

They found that this combination creates improvements in skin wrinkle (crows feet at week 8), skin texture, elasticity and skin texture and it may suggest that astaxanthin used as an oral and a topical supplement may improve skin conditions in all layer

Research (37) - "Efficacy of Astaxanthin for the treatment of Atopic Dermatitis in a Murine Model"

This study investigated whether AST could improve dermatitis and pruritus in a mouse model of Atopic Dermatitis.

To determine the results, there were a number of tests done:
* Behavioural Evaluation;
* Skin Severity Score;
* Serum IgE Level;
* Histological Analyses of Skin; and
* Inflammation Related Factors.

To carry out this study, Astaxanthin (100mg/kg) or Vehicle (olive oil) was orally administered once a day and three times a week for 26 days.

They found that the astaxanthin group had significantly lower clinical skin severity scores and there was a greatly reduced level of scratching. Serum IgE was also greatly decreased and the immune reaction to the dermatitis was also significantly decreased. Therefore, they found that astaxanthin improves the dermatitis and pruritus in Atopic Dermatitis because of the regulation of the inflammatory effects and the expression of inflammatory cytokines.

Research (38) - "Effects of Astaxanthin on dinitrofluorobenzene - induced contact dermatitis in mice"

In this study they investigated potential applications of astaxanthin aside from its antioxidative and antitumor properties.

They found that astaxanthin exhibited anti-allergic and anti-inflammatory effects in a dinitrofluorobenzene induced contact dermatitis mouse model. The topical application inhibited the enlargement of ear thickness or weight gain, which are common side effects of DNFB. It also inhibited inflammatory hyperplasia, oedema, spongiosis and the infiltration of mononuclear cells/mast cells in the ear tissue. This data suggests that that astaxanthin may be useful for treating patients with allergic skin diseases through a mechanism that may be associated with it's anti-inflammatory and anti-allergic activities.

Chapter #20 - Sun Protection

****

Living in Australia I grew up hearing the quote "Slip, Slop, Slap" on a daily basis. Slip on a shirt, slop on the sunscreen and slap on a hat. We have been told that sun will cause skin cancer, that you shouldn't go out in the sun between 9am and 3pm and that you must heavily cover yourself with sunscreen so as to protect yourself. This message has been so overdone in Australia that we are now one of the most Vitamin D deficient countries, even with all the wonderful sun we have.

Not only is sunscreen full of chemicals that are carcinogenic (cancer causing) itself, but it also only blocks the part of the sun that is required for Vitamin D production while the part of the sun that is supposed to cause skin cancer is not blocked. It doesn't make much sense does it.

Well, we now have some good news. Studies have now shown that this amazing antioxidant is able to rejuvenate the skin from deep down within. Although astaxanthin is distributed throughout all the organs within the body, it predominantly accumulates in all of the layers of the skin (whilst sunscreen only covers the top layer). Because of this, it has a remarkable ability to protect against UV radiation, and therefore skin cancer, without the harmful effects of sunscreen.

So, I guess you are asking how it does this. The answer lies within the protective mechanism that the Haematococcus Pluvialis has to have in order to protect itself from the sun. By eating the source of astaxanthin you then begin to create your own internal sunscreen.

However, not only does it protect against skin cancer it also protects you against skin damage. It has been shown that excessive UV radiation can cause sagging skin and wrinkles as well, which studies have shown are prevented when taking astaxanthin.

Recommended Dosage

It is recommended that you take 4mg of astaxanthin daily for two weeks in order to prevent sunburn.

Research (39) - "Vitamin A Status and Metabolism of Cutaneous Polyamines in the Hairless Mouse after UV irradiation: action of beta-carotene and astaxanthin"

In this study, hairless mice were fed various combinations of astaxanthin, beta carotene and retinol for a period of 4 months. * They found that after irradiation, astaxanthin alone or in combination with retinol was substantially effective in preventing photo-ageing of the skin.

Research (40) - "Modulation of UVA light-induced oxidative stress by B-carotene, Lutein and Astaxanthin in cultured fibroblasts"

In this study, they set out to determine the protective effects against UVA induced oxidative stress with 3 different antioxidants - Beta Carotene, Lutein and Astaxanthin. They subjected rat kidney fibroblasts with high doses of UVA light and then they determined which antioxidant was the most protective. * They found that all antioxidants were protective, with astaxanthin producing superior results.

Research (41) - "Modulatory effects of an algal extract containing astaxanthin on UVA-irradiated cells in culture"

In this study they examined the ability of astaxanthin to protect against UVA induced DNA alterations within human skin fibroblasts, human melanocytes and human intestinal CaCo-2 cells. Synthetic astaxanthin was compared with the algal extract (containing astaxanthin). * Results showed that synthetic astaxanthin prevented UVA induced DNA damage at all concentrations. It also prevented DNA damage in melanocytes and intestines. The algal extract displayed protection against UVA induced damage when 10 uM was administered, but not at the lower dosages (10nM or 100 nM).

****

SECTION 3 - ADDITIONAL CONTENT...

****

Chapter #21 - Astaxanthin for Pets

****

For those pet lovers out there, I have some good news for you. Astaxanthin is not just for you, but it has also been proven to be exceptionally helpful for your pets too...

Just like us, your fur child's immune system is of massive importance to how long you have them by your side. From an early age you will find your pet sniffing and eating everything that goes past. I know my dogs do.

Therefore, it is really important that you keep their immune system at full peak so they may fight off any bugs that come their way. However, as your pet ages, their immune function will also decrease and put them at more risk of getting sick.

If possible, you should start looking after their immune system when they are puppies because that is when it is at its fullest potential. This is where astaxanthin comes in super handy.

Studies show that when animals receive supplemental astaxanthin they may experience the following benefits:

- Will help to support their healthy, normal immune response;
- May help to support their cardiovascular health;
- May help to support joint and muscle recovery after exercise;
- Helps support healthy energy function; and
- May help to support their flexibility in movement.

If you are interested in obtaining some for your pet, please go to the section at the end of the book entitled "Where You Can Get It?"...

Research (42) - "Astaxanthin Uptake in Domestic Dogs and Cats"

In this study they set out to investigate the uptake of astaxanthin by plasma, lipoproteins and leukocytes in both dogs and cats.

To do this, they dosed mature female beagle dogs with 0, 0.1, 0.5, 2.5, 10 and 40mg of astaxanthin and then blood was taken at 0, 3, 6, 9, 12 and 24 hours post treatment. They also dosed mature domestic short haired cats with a single dose of 0, 0.02, 0.08, 0.4, 2, 5 and 10 mg astaxanthin and blood was taken at the same interval.

They found that both cats and dogs absorb astaxanthin from their diet. Maximal astaxanthin concentration in the blood was 0.14 mumol/L in both species and was observed at 6-hour post dosing. Astaxanthin was still found in the blood after 24 hours.

They found astaxanthin was mainly associated with higher levels of HDL cholesterol (good cholesterol) but there was also some astaxanthin found within the leukocytes.

Research (43) - "Dietary Astaxanthin enhances immune response in dogs"

Once again, female beagle dogs were fed 0, 10, 20 and 40 mg astaxanthin daily and blood sampled on weeks 0, 6 , 12 and 16 for assessing lymphoproliferation, leukocyte subpopulations, natural killer cell cytotoxicity and concentrations of blood astaxanthin, IgG, IgMand acute phase proteins.

They found that astaxanthin increased the immune response to vaccines, as well as increased the concentrations of IgG, IgM and B Cells. Plasma levels of C Reactive Protein was also lower in the astaxanthin fed dogs, as was the DNA damage and inflammation.

Chapter #22 - Summary Checklist

****

- Incorporate as many astaxanthin rich foods as possible.

- Do not overexercise - Going to extremes when it comes to exercise causes a greater production of free radicals, and therefore more antioxidants will be required.

- Ensure you take the astaxanthin with healthy fats as it is a fat-soluble antioxidant and will not be absorbed otherwise.

- Reduce your alcohol consumption.

- Give up smoking or minimise the amount of cigarette smoke you are around.

- Eat a healthy diet with plenty of nutritious, fresh, antioxidant rich foods.

- Heal Your Gut from any possibly Leaky Gut Syndrome you may be experiencing. This will allow you to absorb these nutrients more readily.

- Remember that it can take 30+ days for it to begin working. Do not give up - it just takes time...

Conclusion

****

So, firstly I want to thank you for reading through to the end of the book. I am hoping by now that you are convinced how beneficial astaxanthin can be on you reaching optimal health. As it is an incredibly safe supplement to take, it may be worth implementing.

If you are suffering from any of the conditions listed or you are lacking in energy and would just like to feel better, then seriously consider giving astaxanthin a go.

Where You Can Get It...

If you are looking for somewhere to find your astaxanthin supplement that is able to be shipped anywhere in the world then you can go to:

http://www.asknaturopathjen.com/store

Testimonials

So, what are you waiting for? Get yourself some astaxanthin and see how great you can feel. Once you have tried it please email me at jen@asknaturopathjen.com and give me a testimonial on how it has helped you. This would be awesome!!!

Once again, thanks very much for reading my book. If you would like to check out the references associated with this e-book, please see below. I have spent a lot of time and effort researching all the information I have given, and I hope it has given you some insight into Healing With Astaxanthin.

****

SECTION 4 – REFERENCES

****

Scientific References

****

1. Mahmoudd FF et al, "In Vitro suppression of lymphocyte activation in patients with seasonal allergic rhinitis and pollen related asthma by cetirizine or azelastine in combination with ginkgolide B or astaxanthin", Acta Physiologica Hungarica, 2012.

2. Haines DD et al, "Summative Interaction between Astaxanthin, Ginkgo Biloba extract and Vitamin C in suppression of respiratory inflammation: a comparison with ibuoprofen", Phytotherapy Research, 2011.

3. Li J et al, "Protective effects of astaxanthin on ConA-induced autoimmune hepatitis by the JNK/p-JNK pathway-mediated inhibition of autophagy and apoptosis", PLoS One, 2015.

4. Miyachi M et al, "Anti-Inflammatory effects of astaxanthin in the human gingival keratinocyte line NDUSD-1", Journal of Clinical Biochemical Nutrition, 2015.

5. Yamada T et al, "Evaluation of therapeutic effects of astaxanthin on impairments in salivary secretion", Journal of Clinical Biochemistry and Nutrition, 2010.

6. Anderson ML, "A Preliminary investigation of the enzymatic inhibition of 5 alpha reduction and growth of prostatic carcinoma cell line LNCap-FGC by natural astaxanthin and saw palmetto in vitro", Journal of Herbal Pharmacotherapy, 2005.

7. Monroy-Ruiz J et al, "Astaxanthin-enriched diet reduces blood pressure and improves cardiovascular parameters in spontaneously hypertensive rats", Pharmacological Research, 2011.

8. Preuss HG et al, "High Dose Astaxanthin lowers blood pressure and increases insulin sensitivity in rats: are these effects interdependent?", International Journal of Medical Sciences, 2011.

9. Al-Amin MM et al, "Astaxanthin improves behavioral disorder and oxidative stress in prenatal valproic acid induced mice model of autism", Behavioral Brain Research, 2015.

10. Yook JS et al, "Astaxanthin supplementation enhances adult hippocampal neurogenesis and spatial memory in mice", Molecular Nutrition and Food Research, 2016.

11. Zhang X et al, Impact of astaxanthin-enriched algal powder of Haematococcus pluvialis on memory improvement in BALB/c mice, Environmental Geochemistry and Health, 2007.

12. Hui Shen et al, Astaxanthin reduces ischemic brain injury in adult rats, FASEB, 2009.

13. Chew BP et al, "A comparison of the anticancer activities of dietary beta carotene, canthaxanthin and astaxanthin in mice in vivo", Anticancer Research, 1999.

14. Ponnuraj Nagendra Prabhu et al, "Antioxidative and Antiproliferative effects of astaxanthin during the initiation stages of 1,2-dimethyl hydrazine induced experimental colon carcinogenesis", Fundamental and Clinical Pharmacology, 2009.

15. Zhang X et al, Carotenoids inhibit proliferation and regulate expression of peroxisome proliferators-activated receptor gamma (PPARy) in K562 cancer cells, Archives of Biochemistry and Biophysics, 2011.

16. Ryu SK et al, "Effect of an oral astaxanthin pro drug (CDX-085) on lipoprotein levels and progression of atherosclerosis in LDLR (-/-) and ApoE (-/-) mice.

17. Ishiki M et al, "Impact of divergent effects of astaxanthin on insulin signaling in L6 cells", Endocrinology, 2013.

18. Bhuvaneswari S et al, "Astaxanthin prevents loss of insulin signaling and improves glucose metabolism in liver of insulin resistant mice", Canadian Journal of Physiology and Pharmacology, 2012.

19. Uchiyama K et al, "Astaxanthin protects beta-cells against glucose toxicity in diabetic db/db mice", Redox Report, 2002.

20. Bennedsen M et al, Treatment of H Pylori infected mice with antioxidant astaxanthin reduces gastric inflammation, bacterial load and modules cytokine release by splenocytes, Immunology Letters, 1999.

21. Murata K et al, Protective effects of astaxanthin from Paracoccus Carotinifaciens on murine gastric ulcer models, Phytotherapy Research, 2012.

22. Iwasaki Tsuneto et al, Effects of Astaxanthin on Eyestrain Induced by Accommodative Dysfunction, Journal of the Eye, 2006.

23. Nagaki Yasunori et al, The Effect of Astaxanthin on Retinal Capillary Blood Flow in Normal Volunteers, Journal of Clinical Therapeutics and Medicine, 2005.

24. Ishikawa S et al, Effect of Astaxanthin on cataract formation induced by glucocorticoids in the chick embryo, Current Eye Research, 2015.

25. Mayumi Ikeuchi et al, Effects of Astaxanthin Supplementation on Exercise – Induced Fatigue in Mice, Biological and Pharmaceutical Bulletin, 2006.

26. Liu PH et al, The Astaxanthin induced improvement in lipid metabolism during exercise is mediated by a PGC-1a increase in skeletal muscle, Journal of Clinical Biochemistry and Nutrition, 2014.

27. Djordjevic B et al, Effect of Astaxanthin Supplementation on muscle damage and oxidative stress markers in elite young soccer players, Journal of Sports Medicine and Physical Fitness, 2012.

28. Earnest CP et al, Effect of Astaxanthin on cycling time trial performance, International Journal of Sports Medicine, 2011.

29. Aoi W et al, Astaxanthin limits exercise induced skeletal and cardiac muscle damage in mice, Antioxidants and Redox Signaling, 2003.

30. Augusti PR et al, "Effect of Astaxanthin on kidney function impairment and oxidative stress induced by mercuric chloride in rats", Food and Chemical Toxicology, 2008.

31. Guo SX et al, "Astaxanthin attenuates early acute kidney injury following severe burns in rats by ameliorating oxidative stress and mitochondrial-related apoptosis", Marine Drugs, 2015.

32. Ni Y et al, "Astaxanthin prevents and reverses diet-induced insulin resistance and steatohepatitis in mice: A comparison with Vitamin E", Scientific Reports, 2015.

33. Kuedo Z et al, "Effects of Astaxanthin from Litopenaeus Vannamei on Carrageenan-Induced Edema and Pain Behavior in Mice", Molecules, 2016.

34. Murata K et al, "Protective Effects of Astaxanthin from Paracoccus Carotinifaciens on Murine Gastric Ulcer Models", Phytotherapy Research, 2012.

35. Yang O et al, Therapeutic Effect of Astaxanthin on acetic-acid-induced gastric ulcers in rats, Europe PMC, 2009.

36. Tominaga K et al, "Cosmetic Benefits of astaxanthin on human subjects", Acta Biochimica Polonica, 2012.

37. Yoshihisa Y et al, "Efficacy of Astaxanthin for the Treatment of Atopic Dermatitis in a Murine Model", PLoS One, 2016.

38. Kim H et al, "Effects of astaxanthin on dinitrofluorobenze - induced contact dermatitis in mice", Molecular Medicine Reports, 2015.

39. Savoure N et al, Vitamin A status and metabolism of cutaneous polyamines in the hairless mouse after UV irradiation: action of beta carotene and astaxanthin, International Journal for Vitamin and Nutrition Research, 1995.

40. O'Connor I et al, Modulation of UVA light-induced oxidative stress by B-Carotene, Lutein and Astaxanthin in Cultured Fibroblasts, Journal of Dermatological Science, 1998.

41. Lyons N et al, Modulatory effects of an algal extract containing astaxanthin on UVA-irradiated cells in culture, Journal of Dermatologica Science, 2002.

42. Park JS et al, "Astaxanthin uptake in domestic dogs and cats", Nutrition and Metabolism, 2010.

43. Chew BP et al, "Dietary Astaxanthin enhances immune response in dogs", Veterinary Immunology and Immunopathology, 2011.

44. Manabe E et al, "Astaxanthin protects mesangial cells from hyperglycemia-induced oxidative signaling", Journal of Cell Biochemistry, 2008.

45. Park JS et al, "Astaxanthin uptake in domestic dogs and cats", Nutrition and Metabolism, 2010.

46. Chew BP et al, "Dietary Astaxanthin enhances immune response in dogs", Veterinary Immunology and Immunopathology, 2011.

47. Manabe E et al, "Astaxanthin protects mesangial cells from hyperglycemia-induced oxidative signaling", Journal of Cell Biochemistry, 2008.

48. Yeh PT et al, "Astaxanthin Inhibits Expression of Retinal Oxidative Stress and Inflammatory Mediators in Streptozotocin-Induced DIabetic Rats", PLoS One, 2016.

49. Li X et al, "Astaxanthin reduces type 2 diabetic-associated cognitive decline in rats via activation of PI3K/Akt and attenuation of oxidative stress", Molecular Medicine Reports, 2016.

50. Ying CJ et al, "Anti-inflammatory Effect of Astaxanthin on the Sickness Behavior Induced by Diabetes Mellitus", Cellular and Molecular Neurobiology, 2015.

51. Lecomte E et al, "Effect of alcohol consumption on blood antioxidant nutrients and oxidative stress indicators", American Journal of Clinical Nutrition, 1994.

Website References

****

- https://uncutwellness.com/astaxanthin-and-autoimmune-disease/

- http://www.lifeextension.com/Protocols/Immune-Connective-Joint/ Autoimmune-Diseases/Page-03

- http://www.lifeextension.com/Protocols/Immune-Connective-Joint/ Autoimmune-Diseases/Page-04

- https://www.andrologyaustralia.org/prostate-problems/prostate-enlargement-or-bph/

- http://www.mayoclinic.org/diseases-conditions/benign-prostatic-hyperplasia/basics/causes/con-20030812

- http://www.mayoclinic.org/diseases-conditions/benign-prostatic-hyperplasia/basics/risk-factors/con-20030812

- http://www.invitehealth.com/both-saw-palmetto-astaxanthin-are-beneficial-for-prostate-prostate-cancer/radio/2006/02/

- http://www.bloodpressureuk.org/BloodPressureandyou /Thebasics/bloodpressure

- http://www.heart.org/HEARTORG/Conditions/High BloodPressure/ SymptomsDiagnosisMonitoringofHighBloodPressure/ What-are-the-Symptoms-of-High-Blood-Pressure_UCM_301871_Article.jsp#.VzK1 atR941I

- http://www.webmd.com/hypertension-high-bloodpressure/guide/blood-pressure-causes

- http://www.resperate.com/medications-and-side-effects/nitric-oxide-your-natural-guard-against-hypertension

- http://care.diabetesjournals.org/content/31/Supplement_2/S181.full

- http://articles.mercola.com/sites/articles/archive/2011/05/14/astaxanthin-the-worlds-strongest-antioxidant.aspx

- http://www.getprograde.com/astaxanthin-and-brain-health.ht ml

- http://naturalsociety.com/antioxidant-astaxanthin-fights-stomach-ulcers/

- https://www.kaahe.org/health/en/273-antioxidants/all.html

- http://www.astaxanthin.co.nz/

- http://medical-dictionary.thefreedictionary.com/Inflammation

- http://healingthebody.ca/astaxanthin-the-ultimate-anti-inflammatory-antiaging-nutrient/

- http://draxe.com/anti-inflammatory-foods/

- http://www.liveinthenow.com/article/anti-inflammatory-supplements-10-that-really-work

- http://products.mercola.com/healthypets/pet-astaxanthin/

- http://www.naturalmedicinejournal.com/journal/2012-02/astaxanthin-review-literature

- http://www.naturalnews.com/041195_pain_relief_supplements_ painkillers.html

- http://www.healthcentral.com/encyclopedia/hc/kidney-diseases-3168920/

- http://www.wholehealthinsider.com/newsletter/nutrient-spotlight-astaxanthin-revisited/

- http://www.mayoclinic.org/diseases-conditions/nonalcoholic-fatty-liver-disease/basics/symptoms/con-20027761

- http://www.mayoclinic.org/diseases-conditions/nonalcoholic-fatty-liver-disease/basics/risk-factors/con-20027761

- http://www.medicinenet.com/script/main/art.asp?articlekey=2
- 951

- http://www.cyanotech.com/pdfs/bioastin/InternalBeauty.pdf

- http://www.diabetes.co.uk/insulin-resistance.html

- http://www.mangomannutrition.com/causes-insulin-resistance-lipid-overload-2/

- http://www.mayoclinic.org/diseases-conditions/arteriosclerosis-atherosclerosis/symptoms-causes/dxc-20167022

- http://www.drwhitaker.com/astaxanthin-benefits-heart-health-inflammation-and-more/

- http://www.cyanotech.com/pdfs/bioastin/batl44.pdf

- http://www.cyanotech.com/pdfs/bioastin/batl43.pdf

- http://www.nutraingredients.com/Research/Study-supports-astaxanthin-s-immune-boosting-power

- http://articles.mercola.com/sites/articles/archive/2012/10/29/a staxanthin-improves-cognitive-function.aspx